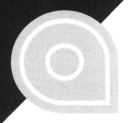

MYplace

FOR DISCOVERY

Published by First Place for Health
Galveston, Texas, USA
www.firstplaceforhealth.com
Printed in the USA
© 2019 First Place for Health

ISBN 978-1-942425-33-5

Caution: The information contained in this book is intended to be solely for informational and educational purposes. It is assumed that the First Place for Health participant will consult a medical or health professional before beginning this or any other weight-loss or physical fitness program.

It is illegal to copy any part of this document without permission of First Place for Health.

All Scripture quotations taken from the Holy Bible, New International Version®, NIV®. Copyright © 1973, 1978, 1984, by Biblica, IncTM. Used by permission of Zondervan Publishing House. All rights reserved worldwide.

Scripture quotations marked ESV are taken from The Holy Bible, English Standard Version® (ESV®) Copyright © 2001 by Crossway, a publishing ministry of Good News Publishers. All rights reserved. ESV Text Edition: 2007

Scripture quotations market NLT are taken from the Holy Bible, New Living Translation, copyright ©1996, 2004, 2007 by Tyndale House Foundation. Used by permission of Tyndale House Publishers, Inc., Carol Stream, Illinois 60188. All rights reserved.

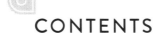

CONTENTS
MY PLACE FOR DISCOVERY: BOOK TWO

My Place for Discovery 4
A Word from the Author 6
About the Author 7

Chapter One
Understanding the *My Place for Discovery* Project 9

Chapter Two
Lost Friendship, Relationship, Love 12

Chapter Three
Lost Possessions 23

Chapter Four
Lost Health 28

Chapter Five
Loss Through Death 33

Chapter Six
Lost Dreams & Opportunities 36

Chapter Seven
Lost Freedom 47

Chapter Eight
Lost Identity 51

Chapter Nine
Lost Job 55

Chapter Ten
Lost Youth 59

Chapter Eleven
Celebration 66

Endnotes 71

MY PLACE FOR DISCOVERY

This book is the second of a four-part series from the First Place for Health wellness program. As you work through these questions and exercises, you will begin to understand your eating and health habits more clearly. Our goal of this series and specifically of book two is to be unafraid as we explore how the losses of our past and present affect our eating habits and weight gain. We want to discover if we have allowed the pain and guilt and grief of loss to sabotage our health. The questions and exercises in this book will guide you through some of life's pain and loss situations so that you can identify any roots of unhealthy behavior.

Loss is a part of life. The cycle of life brings death as new life is created. A seed dies in the ground before becoming a new plant. Leaves and limbs decay, but the result is rich soil for growing. A grandfather lives his life to the full and passes along his legacy to the children who come behind him. Loss doesn't mean we quit or that we are failures. Our goal is to turn loss into a tool to make us stronger. Unfortunately, many of us have reacted to our losses by overfeeding our body.

In modern history, groups such as AA, Celebrate Recovery, Overeaters Anonymous, and others have developed twelve steps to help a person delve into the reasons why he or she chooses alcohol or drugs or food to satisfy deep psychological voids. In the same way, the FP4H *My Place for Discovery Book Two* will help you turn loss into a new perspective and a new focus and a new desire to make right health choices.

While loss may cause some psychological, medical, or personal issues, FP4H does not claim to be doctors, psychologists, or counselors, and we are not equipped to give clinical care to those with deep psychological or medical issues. However, FP4H—and you—have the most powerful tool of all to deal with these and other issues—the Word of God and the power of the Holy Spirit.

The majority of us don't need medical or clinical help—because we have a physical problem with a spiritual answer.

And while we are never against doctors, therapists, or counselors and the good work these professionals do, we know that for most of us, we need spiritual answers. The spiritual expertise we need is found in the Word. So *My Place for Discovery* is written to help you identify what drives you to overeating, and we'll point you in the direction of an answer from God.

Your personal *My Place for Discovery* project centers around four books to be used in conjunction with your FP4H sessions. Each book includes ten lessons. Complete one lesson at a time.

We've kept the *My Place for Discovery* weekly lesson at a practical length so that you will have plenty of time to go deep into your memory, heart, and feelings. One lesson per week will allow plenty of time to work through these personal subjects.

We are excited about the changes that *My Place for Discovery* will make for you.

A WORD FROM THE AUTHOR

I am overweight. It hasn't always been so. In the past, I managed my weight and stayed near the same size—for decades. The weight gain seems to have happened suddenly, and I've failed as I have tried to lose. Now I've been overweight for several years.

When I joined FP4H, I discovered that the weight loss battle is a conflict many others face, too, but I also learned that losing weight is only part of the quest to become healthy. Learning about the four-sided person helped me understand how to live in balance. Understanding how much God cares about my physical body allows me to ask for God's help—a concept I never thought about before joining FP4H. The nutrition lessons and the cooking tips have changed my eating habits. The Bible studies give me strength for the spiritual battles—strength I don't have, if I fight alone. Instead of dwelling on my failures or the scale, my brain is now thinking about healthy foods choices.

But the battle isn't over. My emotions still take control, and I fail. Like you, I worked through the emotional mapping exercises that FP4H provides. As I have studied my emotional mapping charts, I found the trigger that began my journey to overweight. The loss of my job.

I was an executive with great responsibilities and perks. I traveled the world, met heads of state, and negotiated million-dollar deals. I felt accomplished and happy in that position. I began to develop my identity as "corporate Karen." Then, new owners bought the company and eliminated my job. The loss was painful. Financially we were forced to make big lifestyle changes. Physically, we downsized the house, and I no longer got dressed up every day to go to work. Emotionally, I lost my identity as the girl who had made it in a male-dominated business environment. Loss turned my world upside down and made me miserable. I soothed my pain with food.

In our first *My Place for Discovery* book, we discovered some of the reasons we turn to food. That book changed me forever in a spectacular way. In that book, we took a new look at our assets and flaws and considered underlying feelings of selfishness, anger, and negativity that we didn't know were hidden. I caught a glimpse of my love for sugar and then faced it—as a full-blown addiction. It seemed as if sugar controlled my mind and my cravings. If there were cookies in the house, I couldn't resist. If the freezer contained ice cream or the candy jar was filled with candy, I ate until it was gone, whether I was hungry or not. I wanted sweets of all kinds, shapes, and flavors. I satisfied my addiction by sneaking a bite or more when I thought no one was looking. Then, through those exercises in book one, God changed me dramatically. Now I do not crave sweets. I can't describe this incredible change in me except to declare that God has done a miracle. I've lost twenty pounds but the change is much greater than a lower number on the scale. And sugar no longer controls me.

So as we begin book two, I am celebrating. And I am praying that God will intervene again in my life and yours, too. This time, let's ask Him to turn our losses into gains—but not weight gain. Let's ask Him to perform miracles, turning our losses into springboards to health. I can hardly wait to discover what He will do this time.

None of the questions or exercises in this *My Place for Discovery* book are meant to make you hate yourself or to push you deeper into poor behavior. Our goal is to discover the functional and dysfunctional behaviors that are the key to our eating issues.

Let's pray as David prayed, "O Lord, search me."

Karen Porter

ABOUT THE AUTHOR

Karen Porter is a national and international speaker and the author of six books including *Speak Like Jesus* and *I'll Bring the Chocolate* and her latest, *If you Give a Girl a Giant*.

Karen is the founder of kae Creative Solutions, a communications consulting firm and the co-owner of Bold Vision Books, a traditional publishing company. She coaches aspiring writers and speakers and teaches on the national staff of CLASSeminars. She serves on the Board of Directors for several non-profit organizations such as CLASSeminars, First Place for Health, and Advanced Writers and Speakers Association.

Karen considers her marriage to George as her greatest achievement. In her spare time, she continues her life-long quest to find the perfect purse.

CHAPTER ONE: UNDERSTANDING THE *MY PLACE FOR DISCOVERY* PROJECT

Jesus mentioned four distinct spheres of life in Luke 20:27—spiritual, emotional, mental, and physical. FP4H helps each of us find balance within each area as well as a balance of all four areas. We dig into Bible studies, strengthen our minds with memorization, study nutrition, and develop exercise routines. We have also worked on our emotional issues, identifying trigger foods and situations. Many have won the battle with obesity forever; others have begun the journey. But some are stuck on the road to health and freedom.

The percentage of people in the FP4H program who lose weight and keep it off is higher than the general population, but we don't have 100% success. FP4H has been asking why. We believe that living a balanced life—mentally, physically, emotionally, and spiritually is the key. We believe that our program is a Live It plan rather than a fad diet, and we know that it is possible to live in freedom for the rest of our life. So why do we still fight the battle, especially in the area of food choices and weight? FP4H author, Gari Meacham says,

"For too long we've tried to fight a battle with forks that can only be fought with faith." Our battle is not physical, it is spiritual.

Often our battles are found in the depth of our being. We haven't taken the time nor have we had the tools we needed to search deeply or truly understood how our life-altering situations have affected our desire to eat. *My Place for Discovery* is the tool that will help us take a fearless moral inventory to discover the source of the battle.

Read the two sections at the beginning of this book: "Welcome" and "A

Word from the Author." Describe how the first *My Place for Discovery* book affected you.

_____

_____

In book one, we listed some problem areas of our life. We were unafraid as we tried to discover how those struggles affected our eating habits. And then, we searched for solutions in the Word of God. In book two, we are jumping into the effects of loss. Our world can quickly become an unfamiliar place when we face loss. Emotionally, we might feel as if we are going crazy. Mentally, we may feel confused or disconnected. Physically, we are likely to respond by starving or over eating. Spiritually, we may wonder why God hasn't intervened.

You may not want to go back to thinking about or analyzing your losses, but being healthy requires you to review and perhaps dismantle what happened so that you can move on. An ancient proverb says, "To make an omelet you have to break a few eggs." Examining our losses bravely and understanding how much God loves us through our losses is our goal in *My Place for Discovery - Book Two*.

The battle for freedom is why FP4H has developed the *My Place for Discovery* project. Although physiologists and psychologists have reviewed and approved the FP4H program, we do not seek to offer solutions from the medical or psychology realm. Emotions and feelings don't always reflect external reality; instead they reflect our internal reality. We believe we have a physical problem with a spiritual solution. Some issues cannot be perceived by the five senses because they are only seen through the Holy Spirit's eyes. At FP4H our expertise is spiritual, because we have the Word of God, which gives us answers to our dilemma.

All Scripture is breathed out by God and profitable for teaching, for reproof, for correction, and for training in righteousness, that the man of God may be complete, equipped for every good work (2 Timothy 3:16).

Our power comes from God.

So let's begin searching for those difficulties that keep us from accessing His power in our health pursuits.

This book contains one lesson for each week of your FP4H session. It is a supplement and a companion to your Bible study. Work through one each week and be ready to discuss the lesson in your FP4H class meeting.

CHAPTER TWO: LOST FRIENDSHIP, RELATIONSHIP, LOVE

We are built to be relational people. We have a basic human prerequisite for contact and connection. God embedded us with a necessity for friendships and relationships. In short, we need each other.

Friendship
In the space below, write the names of your childhood friends. Beside each name, describe how you knew each other (Example: Janie from the neighborhood or Mike, a family friend or Kathy, a school friend) and then note why you were friends (Example: you liked the same sports or music or activities.) Write a short sentence describing something that you and this friend did together (Example: We shared rides to school each day or we went to the same church.)

1. _____

2. _____

3. _____

In the space below, write the names of your teenage and college age friends. Beside each name, describe how you knew each other and why you were friends Write a short sentence describing something that you and this friend did together

1. _____

2. _____

3. _____

In the space below, write the names of your adult friends. Beside each name, describe how you know each other (Example: from work, church, family) and why your friendship blossomed (Example: you like the same sports or music or activities.). Describe at least one activity that you do or did together.

1. _____

2. _____

3. _____

Now pick one friend from each group, whose friendship is not close anymore. Describe why you are no longer connected to that friend. (Example: moved away, move in different circles now, a misunderstanding, a hurtful situation).

1. **<u>Childhood</u>**_____

2. **<u>Teen</u>**_____

3. **<u>Adult</u>**_____

How do the losses of these friendships make you feel?

_____

_____

As you think of any awkward or hurtful events surrounding the loss of one of your friends, consider how you've handled the loss. Have you reconciled any bad feelings in your mind? Describe how or how not.

_____

_____

_____

Have you sought forgiveness or tried to mend any hurts between the two of you? If so, how did your efforts workout? If not, describe why the relationship wasn't mended.

_____

_____

_____

_____

How has the loss of friendship affected your eating habits? (Be honest here about emotional eating.)

_____

_____

_____

_____

A friendship in turmoil brings us to a low place in our emotions and the consequences of unresolved pain are real. In fact, the anguish of lost friendships rips at our core, attacking our self-esteem and identity in Christ.

Relationships and Love
Do you remember your first love? If so, write the person's name in the space below.

_____

_____

Some of us will have one of those stories about how they met their life-long partner in elementary school. For most of us, what we thought was love in junior high, high school, or young adulthood may have been infatuation and not true love. Even so, when that "love" was lost, we can vouch for the fact that the break-up was painful. What is your relationship with your "first love" today? Does remembering him or her cause you any pain or anxiety?

_____

_____

Loss of relationship is one of the most common tools of our Enemy. He will use anything to destroy us and will even dig up feelings from long-ago lost relationships to torture us. According to John 15:11, what is God's plan for our lives?

_____

_____

Does this plan and desire of God apply even when we feel sad, lonely, rejected, or abandoned? Explain.

_____

_____

_____

Read John 15:9 and Psalm 136:26. What is God's feeling toward us? Now read John 15:13 and 15. How is Jesus' relationship with us described? How does knowing this about Jesus make you feel?

_____

_____

Loss of friendships and relationships (especially love relationships) produces negative reactions in us. In the list below, check any attitudes that you have felt or actions you have taken as a result of your lost friendship or love.

_____Rebellion against parent or the church
_____Fear of future friendships or relationships
_____Pretend I'm strong
_____Isolation. Why get involved; I'll just get hurt!
_____Blame God
_____Over activity
_____Suspicious of every potential friend or relationship
_____Feel sorry for myself
_____Feel worthless
_____Feel hopeless
_____Jealous of others

Christ loves us and created us to love others. Read Matthew 22:37-39 and Romans 12:10. Using the two columns below, list specific ways that you love others and specific actions you could take to become a better friend.

Love Actions I Take	Loves Actions I Need to Take

Identify your "people" losses. In the chart below, list the name of a friend, a relationship, or a love, and then identify the cause of the loss. For example, I might list my friend Mary. We were close but now we rarely speak or connect with each other, partially because I moved away, but also because I never tried to keep the connections alive. Or I might list my friend Peg who I felt wasn't loyal to me in a tough situation. After listing the name and the cause, list your feelings about this loss and how you have reacted to it in relation to food.

Relationship	The Cause	My Mistake	My Feelings	Related to Food

Whether it is a close acquaintance, a romance, or a long-time friendship, losing a relationship hurts. Confusion about what happened to the relationship mingles with the wound and then, feelings of anger or self-righteousness surface. We assign fault, face grief, and feel sadness.

Choose one of the individuals listed in the previous chart. Write the person's name in the space below. Answer the following questions about that person.

_____

Describe the person and then circle all the descriptions that apply.

Solid	Inconsistent	Lively
Temperamental	Unpredictable	Happy
Funny	Strong	Needy
Selfish	Giving	Gloomy
Quiet	Talkative	Outgoing
Withdrawn	Overpowering	Silly

As you consider the experience of losing this friendship or relationship, examine your feelings related to that loss. Circle all that apply.

Sadness	Ready to scream	Disappointment
Revenge	Tears	Withdrawal
Lonely	Bitter	Out of Control
Humiliated	Anger	Blame
Grief	Confusion	Responsibility

What is your behavior related to the loss? What is the least wise decision you've made when you think of that person or as you have tried to get over the loss of this friendship? Check all that apply.

- ☐ Eat Ice Cream
- ☐ Shop
- ☐ Take a trip on the credit card
- ☐ Write him or her off and try to forget them
- ☐ Turn to a destructive relationship
- ☐ Regret
- ☐ Overeat
- ☐ Binge on salty foods
- ☐ Try to make the former friend jealous
- ☐ Go on a twitter or FB rampage against the person
- ☐ _____

One of the wisest decisions we can make about lost friendships is to think through our personal role in the loss. Be bold as you mark the list below. Check all that apply.

- ☐ Was I too busy to see what might happen?
- ☐ Was I too proud to reach out to my friend?
- ☐ Did I always want my way in the friendship?
- ☐ Was I constantly trying to impress this person?
- ☐ Did I secretly think unkind thoughts about my friend or judge his or her actions?
- ☐ Was I a loyal friend?
- ☐ Other _____

You may never know why your friend let you down but you will feel the impact of the lost friendship in ways you didn't expect. You'll remember her birthday, but not acknowledge it to her. You'll think of him when something big happens, and you'll wish you could tell him. You'll hear a funny joke that you know she'd laugh at, but you don't call. You'll struggle with whether to blame him, and there will be days you'll be so happy that you don't have to talk to him.

It is important to dismantle whatever myths you've told yourself about losing the relationship—because your health depends on it. Even the best friend cannot change you, heal your wounds, or fix your pain. Answering these questions will help.

1. What expectations did I have for the relationship, and what did that relationship give me?

   _____

   _____

2. What good features will I keep from that relationship as I move forward?

   _____

   _____

3. What damaging features from that relationship will I leave behind as I move forward?

   _____

   _____

4. How has the loss of this relationship changed my healthy food choices in a negative or positive way? Please explain your answer.

   _____

   _____

Healthy Moving On
We process the grief of loss in different ways depending on our personality type and our personal relationship with God. There are some steps we can

take to heal in a healthy way.

Write a letter to the person (but don't send it)
It isn't healthy to "have your last say" and tell the person off if you really send the letter, but it may be helpful to write your feelings and then, (and this is important) shred the letter. Begin by reflecting on the relationship when it was good. Continue by writing about how you felt betrayed or abandoned. Then write out your plan for a healthy future—new choices, clean foods, exercise, new activities, and new friends.

Respond with kindness
Though you think revenge would feel good, read what the Bible says in Ephesians 4:31-32. List what we should do instead of bitterness, wrath, anger, and slander.

_____

_____

_____

Consider how you will choose to respond gently and generously. List several specific actions below. For example, send a gift or a nice card. Call the friend. Say something nice about the friend to someone else.

_____

_____

_____

Balance
To move on, find a resolution in all the areas of the four-sided person. Physically, if seeing that person causes you pain, plan your activities so

that you can avoid contact. Don't follow him or her on social media. Mentally, rethink the causes for the loss of this relationship and accept that the person may never tell you why. Emotionally, reach out to others for a new sense of connection. Volunteer to serve your community. Spiritually, turn to Christ by spending time alone with Him and reading His Word. Above all, make healthy eating and exercising your priority as you heal.

In the space below, make a plan of how you will stay balanced in each of the four areas:

Physically _____

Mentally _____

Emotionally _____

Spiritually _____

Reflect
In the space below, write your thoughts about friendship, listing what you desire in a good friend or special relationship. Be honest about potentially bad choices you could make and the possibility that you might grasp at friendship for fear of being alone. Ask God to help you become a good friend and to find relationships that will honor him.

_____

_____

_____

CHAPTER THREE: LOST POSSESSIONS

When we have lost property, money, and belongings due to storms, schemes, hacks, or mistakes, we feel the damage. And if the loss is because of some injustice, such as a theft, we feel violated.

A teenager worked hard, saving her money for a trip to a resort with her family only to have a pickpocket take it all. A new car is crushed in an accident. A husband and wife crouch in a bathtub listening to the terrifying winds of a tornado as it touches down on their house. An irreplaceable, precious family heirloom is lost in a residential fire. A laptop or tablet is left on a plane and never found. Losing possessions and property is a painful and tragic circumstance. The teenager's disappointment and feeling of violation turned a joy-full trip into sadness. The car owner never feels good about the car even after it is repaired. The couple experiences fear and horrific damage. The loss of the nostalgic item breaks hearts, and the loss of the technology tool leaves the owner feeling useless. If we aren't careful, we will be overwhelmed and the loss will lead us to unhealthy living.

In her book, *Food, Faith, and Finish Lines*, Joyce Ainsworth tells the story about how a loss almost sent her back to her old eating habits.

> A second surprise detour rocked my world when a tornado ripped through Magee, Mississippi. My precious parents, both in their seventies, had already weathered Hurricane Katrina a few years prior. Now an EF3 tornado struck the north part of their city. The tornado significantly damaged the town's water treatment plant, interrupting service to the entire town. The tornado also destroyed sixty homes. One of those homes belonged to my parents.
>
> They lost much that day, but were blessed to be alive. The physical destruction was overwhelming but the emotional devastation was the real detour for me. I sat in their front yard and ate a gallon-size bag of homemade chocolate chip cookies. One cookie was not enough. I cried, ate a cookie, cried, ate a cookie, cried some more, until I was totally emotionally spent.

Joyce's weight loss story is a magnificent example of what God can do, but even after months and years of making healthy food choices, the tragedy of her family's loss almost sent Joyce back to her bad eating habits without thinking.

Until she saw the empty bag.

Imagine working as hard as Joyce to lose weight and having the kind of success she had, and then reverting to the comfort of sugar without thinking. In her case, the loss was her parent's loss, but the pain drove her back to former eating habits. Loss is a powerful influence on us.
  Truth is, we have all been there with her. We are weak. But God offers freedom and victory.

In the space below, list a possession that you have lost and the circumstances that led to that loss.

Possession	Circumstance

If the loss was due to an accident or storm or fire or something else out of your control, describe the damage and cost.

_____

_____

_____

_____

Did you have any of the following physical responses to the event?

Circle all that apply.

Stomach ache	Dizziness
Irregular breathing	Racing Heart Rate
Feeling faint	Trembling

Other _____

These and other physical reactions are probably normal, but if they don't go away and you become frightened by your reaction, it might be time to talk to a medical professional.

Sometimes the emotional damage of trauma is more devastating than the actual loss. Describe your emotions as you faced the loss using the following chart.

Circle all that apply.

Distress	Loss of hope	Grief
Loss of security	Shock	Anger
Depression	Disbelief	Stressed
Inconsolable	Nightmares	Feeling Numb
Confused	Helpless	

No one who experiences a disaster is untouched by the experience. But as First Place for Health member and award winning author, Cynthia Ruchti, says, "Don't judge your final outcome by the first walk-through of the storm damage." After the initial reactions, you should be able to think clearly and make plans for your future after the loss. To help you determine if you are dwelling on the loss, write a paragraph describing how you feel about the loss today.

_____

_____

_____

It is possible that your traumatic loss has so stressed you emotionally that you need to see a professional counselor. You may be the last person to recognize your reaction or possible PTSD. While there is no exact way we should respond to stress, each of us needs to evaluate our reactions if we feel overwhelmed, especially if we can't think clearly.

Joyce says, "I had heard of people falling off the wagon, but I was not only off the wagon, I was knee-deep in mud. But God knew where I was, and after the emotional detour of wind, cookies, and tears, He reached down and loved me, mud and all."

You may never forget the pain of your loss or the stress related to it, but with God's help, you can move forward with new goals, dreams, focus, and freedom. When you do, you will change your future, change your life, and change your results. In the spaces below, write some lofty goals for your new reality.

Physical Goals
Eating. (Vegetables, lean meat, low fat dairy will give you energy ard endurance and if you lose weight, you will feel more confident and positive.) Write your goal in the space below.

_____

_____

Exercise. (Exercising releases good endorphins to boost your energy and if you are purposeful in planning your exercise, you may reduce that "stuck" feeling that keeps you from moving on from the traumatic event.) Write your goal in the space below.

_____

_____

_____

Mental. (Memorizing Scripture will burn the Word of God into your mind, and then when you feel stressed or depressed, the powerful all-healing words will give you comfort and peace.) Write your goal in the space below.

_____

_____

_____

Emotional. (Beginning a gratitude list will help you build a God-perspective on your feelings and when your emotions threaten to drag you down, you will find joy in being thankful for life.) Write your goal in the space below.

_____

_____

_____

CHAPTER FOUR: LOST HEALTH

I have a friend who is a great Bible teacher and a vibrant man of God. A few years ago, he contracted a devastating viral disease, which went undiagnosed for many months. Now, even after getting the appropriate treatments and medicine, he is plagued with muscle and leg weakness, uncontrollable shaking, and mental confusion. Today, there is little resemblance to strong man before the disease debilitated him.

I have broken my legs on three different occasions and while I have mostly recovered through surgeries and rehabilitation, the lingering pain, stiffness, and limited mobility have changed my life drastically.

Author and speaker Jennifer Rothschild is blind and has been since she was a teenage girl. She says she has now lived in physical darkness longer than she did in physical light. Blindness changed her life

Have you experienced some illness or loss that has given you new challenges in life? Write about it—no matter how small the loss or the challenge may seem.

_____

_____

_____

How has this life-change affected your healthy food and exercise choices?

_____

_____

_____

Jennifer Rothschild, who we mentioned above says, "Blindness is hard, but it's been a place where God has shown Himself to be so kind strong, and faithful. That's why I do what I do—because God has made it well with my soul." How has God used your lost health to make it well with your soul?

_____

_____

_____

Read Psalm 62:5. What does the verse say about finding rest in God?

_____

_____

_____

How does finding rest in God help you with the health challenges you have experienced?

_____

_____

_____

Read James 1:2-4. Explain how this verse could encourage a person who has health issues.

_____

_____

_____

What does verse 4 say that faith produces in a person who is going through a trial?

_____

_____

_____

How do you define faith?

_____

_____

_____

How do you define endurance?

_____

_____

_____

It is probable that you have handled your personal health challenge or illness with faith sometimes and without faith sometimes. Describe how you feel when you exercise your faith. Then write a few sentences about your experiences when you have doubted and failed to have faith.

_____

_____

_____

We need encouragement when we face illness or loss due to health issues. Listed below are several encouraging quotes about health issues. In the space below each one, write how this quote helps you face your loss. Be honest; if the quote makes you angry or seems impossible, say so.

"Some days there won't be a song in your heart. Sing anyway"...Emory Austin

_____

_____

_____

"The greatest healing therapy is friendship and love." ...Hubert H. Humphrey

_____

_____

_____

"With a new day comes new strength and new thoughts." ...Eleanor Roosevelt

_____

_____

_____

"Even if you have a terminal disease, you don't have to sit down and mope. Enjoy life and challenge the illness that you have." ...Nelson Madela

_____

_____

"Since my illness, I've felt the presence of angels." ...Fran Drescher

_____

_____

_____

"Without anxiety and illness, I would have been a ship without a rudder."
...Edvard Munch

_____

_____

_____

CHAPTER FIVE: LOSS THROUGH DEATH

My friend said, "I wish I could talk to my mom one more time." The loss continues to cause pain. Grief is painful and can overwhelm us with other emotions such as despair (thinking we can't continue to live without the person) and guilt (thinking we should have been kinder or more helpful or understanding or more available). The grief will overwhelm us when we least expect it. A date on the calendar or seeing a view you had shared together. A smell. An event. A word. And grief shows up.

I've felt that pain and grief and guilt, especially when my mother passed away. I finally had to understand that I did the best I could. I've used some tools to help me face the loss and then face my life without the person.

Tool number one: The Words You Speak
Instead of saying, "the day she died," substitute the words, "on her heaven day." Those simple words change loss into joy. What words could you use to help you through your loss?

_____

_____

Tool number two: The Way You Remember
Instead of concentrating on the loss of that person and his or her influence and love in your life, remember something that makes you smile. Write about it here.

_____

_____

_____

Researchers have discovered that we experience grief in various ways. Read over the following lists and mark the experiences you've had during your grief.

Physical Signs

- ☐ Diarrhea
- ☐ Dizziness
- ☐ Fast Heartbeat or Tightness in the Chest
- ☐ Feeling Like There's a Lump in Your Throat
- ☐ Headaches
- ☐ Hyperventilating or Shortness of Breath
- ☐ Loss of Appetite or Weight Loss
- ☐ Nausea
- ☐ Tiredness
- ☐ Trouble Sleeping

Emotional Signs

- ☐ Anger
- ☐ Crying Spells
- ☐ Loneliness
- ☐ Restlessness and Irritability
- ☐ Sadness or Depression

Mental Signs

- ☐ Disorganization and Lack of Concentration
- ☐ Self-blame
- ☐ Sense that What's Happening isn't Real

What sad emotions surface when you think of the loss of this person? Circle as many as apply.

Guilt   Heartbreak   Anger

Unhappy   Lonely

List some ways you can undo the sad emotions, replacing them with joy in remembering and thanksgiving that you had that person in your life.

_____

_____

_____

Now think about your eating habits since the death of your loved one. In the space below, write any insights you have now about how grief may have affected what you eat, when you eat, and how much you eat.

_____

_____

_____

As you look over the paragraph you wrote above about how grief has affected your eating habits, what actions do you need to take now so that your new response will be self-control and healthy eating habits?

_____

_____

_____

CHAPTER SIX: LOST DREAMS AND OPPORTUNITIES

We can't live successfully without dreams. It is part of the human condition that we need to look forward to the future.

Dreams may not come true. And plans will fail. J. K. Rowling, author of the Harry Potter series said this about failure, "It is impossible to live without failing at something, unless you live so cautiously that you might as well not have lived at all—in which case, you fail by default."

God places dreams into the fabric of your life. But if your dream is broken or delayed or feels impossible, it isn't the end of your hope. Winston Churchill said, "Success is not final, failure is not fatal." God will give you a new dream and the new path He gives you will be more magnificent than any dream you ever dreamed before—if you don't quit. Churchill continued, "It is the courage to continue that counts."

How do you think the loss of a dream and the possibility of a new dream affect your health and your First Place journey?

_____

_____

_____

One of the main characters (an older man) in a movie recounted part of the story of his life. He had dreamed of becoming a history professor and was attending community college at night to get his degree. Then his wife became pregnant so the man quit college to get a job to provide for his growing family. He stayed in that job for 45 years. Now that he was older, he wondered what happened to his life. Where was his dream?

Maybe your story follows the same pattern. Great potential and a big dream interrupted by a life reality. Too often we never go back to the dream. Necessity takes the wheel from dreams and aspirations. Using the following prompts, write what your younger self would've said about your dreams.

What were your dreams:

As a child: _____

_____

_____

As a young adult: _____

_____

_____

As you began family life (single or married): _____

_____

_____

Which of these dreams did you accomplish?

_____

_____

What dream did you not reach yet?

_____

_____

Using the words below, describe your feelings about not reaching that dream?

- ☐ Accepted that I may never reach the dream
- ☐ Resignation that I couldn't do it and never will be
- ☐ Anticipation that I will eventually reach the dream
- ☐ What if my dream is replaced with something else?

As you think about your feelings, answer this question: How does the loss or delay of that dream affect your eating?

_____

_____

_____

Describe your reactions:

_____

_____

_____

What choices did you make that stifled the dream?

Job or Career Choices

_____

_____

_____

Relationship Choices

_____

_____

_____

Spiritual Choices

_____

_____

_____

Emotional Choices

_____

_____

_____

Physical Choices

_____

_____

What choice took you down a road you never intended to go down? Explain what happened.

_____

_____

_____

As you look back on these choices and your reactions to the dreams that seem lost, look carefully to discover any pattern regarding your health—especially eating patterns. Write your thoughts.

_____

_____

_____

How do you feel about the dream now? Can you see an opportunity for the dream to be revived? Explain.

_____

_____

_____

Sometimes in life, God allows us to face disappointment and pain especially regarding our well-crafted plans. He even lets a dream die. But, He always comes through with a bigger better dream that will give you great joy. Can you describe how God has blessed you even if your dreams didn't turn out like you expected?

_____

_____

God has planned a great journey for you. You may have taken a few wrong turns such as making bad choices, gaining weight, endangering your health, hurting those you love the most. You know you haven't fulfilled your destiny and you doubt you will ever succeed. God has a plan for your future. (See Jeremiah 33:11.)

Write a prayer below asking God to fill you with enthusiasm for His future plans for you.

_____

_____

_____

Everyone wants to be a success. Yet throughout a person's life, he or she makes decisions that affect the rest of his or her days. Sometimes these decisions are clearly the right decision, and we take the right fork in the road and go happily down our path. Other times, we make a decision that is the wrong direction and we end up in a place we never intended.

Loss is defined as "the state of being without." A deeper look at the meaning also reveals that a definition is "no order or schedule." How do these definitions apply to the losses that we bring on ourselves by not doing what we should have done or by making a poor choice?

_____

_____

Is the loss different because you

- ☐ Didn't know any better
- ☐ Should've known what to do
- ☐ Willfully decided to disobey
- ☐ Were afraid
- ☐ Were not strong

Explain your answer:

When we have lost an opportunity because of our choice or our actions, we often feel guilt. We judge ourselves for our failures and inabilities. Write your personal definition of the following:

Man's judgment

Self-judgment

God's judgment

Now read 1 Corinthians 4:3-4. What does Paul say about judgment?

Judging by some artificial standard or personal preferences or ingrained prejudices isn't fair judgment. The only true basis for judgment is the Word.

Now consider a time when you judged yourself harshly for overeating and describe your feelings and your motives below.

_____

_____

We can evaluate every decision by two fundamental questions about the loss of opportunity. First, how does the loss make you feel? Second, how does your reaction make God feel? Answering those two questions in every situation helps us overcome the losses we have faced and honest answers

When Dawn turned 50, she gave up hope of having a child of her own. Though she and her husband had tried all the medical procedures and had prayed, the opportunity for her to become pregnant was lost.

How do you think Dawn feels?

_____

_____

How do you think Dawn's situation makes God feel?

_____

_____

What choices does Dawn have now?

_____

_____

Roger never finished college. As a young man, he worked hard, learning the business and impressing his bosses. Now after all his hard work, management has hired younger men who don't know the business or the industry as well as Roger does. He knows he will never get the big promotions at work because he doesn't have a college degree.

How do you think Roger feels?

_____

_____

How do you think Roger's situation makes God feel?

_____

_____

Evie attended First Place for Health and found success, losing three dress sizes and lowering her blood sugar and blood pressure. Her church asked her to become a leader in the next fall session. She was excited and pleased. But in her excitement, she lost her focus on eating healthy and gained most of her weight back. She missed her opportunity to become a vibrant leader in the program she loves.

How do you think Evie's situation makes her feel?

_____

_____

How do you think Evie's situation makes God feel?

_____

_____

Each of the people in these examples had choices to make in the wake of losing the opportunity they had dreamed about. Think about some good and bad responses

What would be some unhealthy responses to each of these lost opportunities? Circle one or two and explain why it would be an unhealthy response.

Unhealthy Response:

Food	Sweets	Anger
Shopping	Lashing Out	Ssearching Recipe Books
Gossip	Resentment	

What would be some healthy responses to each of these lost opportunities? Circle one or two and explain why it would be a healthy response.

Healthy Response:

Bible reading	Trust in God	List of New Dreams
Forgiveness	Moving Forward	

Let's consider how we handle loss of opportunity and poor decisions we've made. Circle whether you think each one is a healthy or unhealthy response.

1)	Avoiding painful stimuli such as photos, places, clothing —	Healthy	Unhealthy
2)	Distraction – working too hard	Healthy	Unhealthy
3)	Drug Abuse	Healthy	Unhealthy
4)	Alcohol Abuse	Healthy	Unhealthy
5)	Food Abuse	Healthy	Unhealthy
6)	Moving – getting out of the location of the problem	Healthy	Unhealthy

Do you think God can't bless you because you blew it in the decision you made?

_____

_____

Do you think God will forgive you when you were disobedient? Explain.

_____

_____

Our view of God is crucial as to how we behave and what we will do next when our options are lost. Every response is based on our understanding of God's power over our circumstances, His design for our future, and His love for our soul.

Most of the godly men and women in the Bible failed in some way—some in dramatic and disastrous ways. Perhaps no one in history missed an opportunity more than Peter, who stood by the fire denying that he knew Christ. Yet God gave a second chance. What characteristic of God allows Him to forgive us and give us new opportunities? Read Ephesians 4:7; Hebrews 4:16; and Romans 6:14 and then, write your description of how God treats us when we fail.

_____

_____

Write a prayer thanking God for second chances.

_____

_____

CHAPTER SEVEN: LOST FREEDOM

Freedom is an interesting word and an intriguing concept. We want freedom and yet some of us may not be ready to live in freedom, because we turn freedom on its heels until it becomes permission. Freedom is uncontrolled choices about good food and exercise. Instead, when we turn freedom into permission, we eat whatever we want until we feel miserable. Some of us reject freedom so we have developed a severe and rigid control over the quantity and type of food we eat. We are not free; we have traded one prison for another.

The FP4H plan is well balanced dealing with four areas of life: physical, mental, emotional, and spiritual. The program leads to balanced living which in turn leads to freedom.

Knowing that the FP4H program leads you to freedom, it is time to honestly answer the question, "Are you consciously, consistently and whole-heartedly doing the program?" Before you answer this question, pray. Ask the Lord to help you see your participation in FP4H from His viewpoint. Then write your answer in the space below.

Let's get specific and completely honest with ourselves:

1) Am I tracking every bite?   Yes   No   Sometimes
2) Am I completing the Bible study each day?   Yes   No   Sometimes
3) Am I praying for my prayer partner each day?   Yes   No   Sometimes
4) Am I exercising each day?   Yes   No   Sometimes
5) Am I memorizing the memory verse each week?   Yes   No   Sometimes

Remember that the success of FP4H isn't necessarily about your weight—though we believe weight loss will be valuable to you. The real success measure is whether you are healthier than when you began the program.

Evaluate yourself in the following areas:

Weight – Have you lost weight? Are you working on it? Write your honest thoughts about your success and failures with weight? What do you think leads to victory and what do you think leads to defeat?

_____

_____

Quiet Time – Have you set an unbreakable appointment with the Lord each day? What disciplines are you practicing? Write a description of the place where you meet God each day. Describe how it looks, how it feels, and then describe what you do when you enter into your Quiet Time.

_____

_____

Have you considered some new worship or study techniques (such as using sign language or reading and singing hymns or drawing or coloring) to invigorate your quiet time? Write those below and share with the class.

_____

_____

Changes – Since joining FP4H, have you changed your behavior in the area of food? How?

_____

_____

Exercise? Are you intentionally moving and challenging your body each day?

_____

_____

Prayer? How has your prayer life changed since joining FP4H?

_____

_____

Grocery Shopping? Do you buy more foods from the perimeter of the grocery store now? What food choices have you made? What don't you buy anymore?

_____

_____

Snacks? What food do you keep on hand so that you will be able to snack in a healthy way?

_____

_____

Success? Have you stopped unproductive or destructive behavior?

_____

_____

Reality Check

Have you traded one obsession for another such as shopping, crafts, over exercise, rigorous calorie counting?

_____

_____

If you lived in freedom, how would you live? (Read Galatians 5:13.)

_____

_____

How would you escape the feelings? (Read John 8:36.)

_____

_____

How would you clear your mind? (Read Galatians 5:1.)

_____

_____

How will you heal your heart? (Read 1 Corinthians 6:12.)

_____

_____

Write a prayer in the space below, asking God for genuine freedom.

_____

_____

CHAPTER EIGHT: LOST IDENTITY

Before Jesus' death, Mary poured expensive perfume on His feet. She worshipped Him. She didn't seem to care about the expense of the perfume (perhaps it was her dowry) or the spectacle she made of herself as she let down her hair. She emptied her alabaster box—and she emptied herself.

One of our goals for this second *My Place for Discovery* book is to empty ourselves so we can be filled with the hope and confidence that the Holy Spirit gives to us as believers.

Empty Myself of the Unclean
Recognizing the unclean deep within may be easy for you, like identifying a shriveled cucumber in a fridge drawer. I hope so. But finding the obstacles and barriers caused by bitterness or anger or defeat may take probing and rummaging for some of us. The choice is mine. I can empty out the unclean and start anew.

As you think about emptying yourself of the unclean do any of the ideas below come to your mind?

Movies I Watch	Books I read
Jokes I Listen to	Anger I allow
Bitterness I Hoard	Disobedience I practice
Impatience I Embrace	Food I choose
Hate I Accumulate	Words I say
Hurts I Collect	_____

Empty Myself of the Proud
Each of us possess abilities that are good and admirable. We should celebrate and feel good about our talents and skills—until we cross over into the arena of pride, which is that feeling that my kindness, my goodness, my

brain, my accomplishments, my Bible knowledge, or my spiritual prowess is superior to all others.

Mary had possession of a full pint of nard. It belonged to her. It was valuable and beautiful. She could have held on to it. Instead she emptied it. She gave Him the best she had. We should strive for excellence in all we do and believe in our abilities and skills, but never allow our thoughts to move into prideful, self-serving beliefs.

What about you is good and worthy?

_____

_____

How can you give these qualities over to God so that you won't become prideful in them?

_____

_____

Empty Myself of the Mediocre
Mediocrity is accepting the status quo in any situation. Circle the three words below that best define mediocre in your mind.

Decent	Second-rate	Uninspired
Dull	Colorless	Indifferent
Inferior	Passable	Tolerable
Ordinary	Undistinguished	Medium

Using the three words you circled, describe how these words affect you in the following areas.

Family Relationships

_____

_____

Work Success

_____

_____

Spiritual Growth

_____

_____

Now that you have considered areas where your actions might be below average in family, work, and spiritually, consider what you can do to rise out of mediocrity. Write your thoughts below.

_____

_____

Identity and Pride
Sometimes we allow our abilities or lack of abilities dictate our identity but what you do or can do does not define you. Your weight does not say whether God loves you. If you've failed and feel worthless, these feelings do not define you. If you've been undisciplined with food, the lack of self-control doesn't define you. We stand in the closet hating our clothes and ourselves. Self-rejection leads to self-unforgiveness, self-resentment, and self-hate. God never hates you or rejects you. Each of us must find our lost identity in Christ regardless of how good we've been (pride) or how bad we've been (self-hate).

MYplace ○ FOR DISCOVERY

Read Psalm 139:13-16. How did God make you?

_____

_____

According to verse 16, did your poor choice surprise God? Why?

_____

_____

Read Ephesians 2:10. Who are you in God's eyes?

_____

_____

Do you believe God loves you? In the space below, tell how God has shown you love in the past week? Be ready to share this experience with your group.

_____

_____

CHAPTER NINE: LOST JOB

Losing a job is traumatic whether you expected the downsizing or you were surprised with the news. Your job influences every aspect of your way of life—entertainment, purchases, and lifestyle. Not having the assurance of your paycheck will cause you stress and anxiety. And finding a new job is not always easy. For those who are entrepreneurs or self-employed, losing a big project may generate some of the same feelings.

Have you lost a job or other source of income?

_____

_____

Were you surprised, shocked, or expecting the loss?

_____

_____

How did you react?

_____

_____

Did you find other employment or ways to supplement your income quickly?

_____

_____

How did the loss make your feel about your future?

_____

_____

Some broken dreams are the consequences of our failure to wait on God. In Genesis 12, Sarai got tired of waiting on God. She and Abram had received a promise from God that they would have many descendants, but Sarai never got pregnant. After ten years, Sarai stopped waiting on God. She offered her maid to Abram so there would be a child in the house.

God did not break His promise, He just made them wait. Sarai's impatience made her try to help God keep His promise.

Impatience leads us to make wrong decisions and lose opportunities. From the list below, circle what makes you impatient.

Slow people	Slow Decisions
Ineffective Leaders	Slow Internet
Waiting	On Hold on Phone
Doctor Appointment	Standing in Line
Water to Boil	Trailers at Movies
Slow Restaurant	Unanswered Emails
Slow Fast Food Window	Boredom
Copy Machines	Bus or Train off Schedule
Meeting too Long	Meeting off Agenda

"The demand for instant results is seeping into every corner of our lives, and not just virtually. Retailers are jumping into same-day delivery services. Smartphone apps eliminate the wait for a cab, a date, or a table at a hot restaurant. Movies and TV shows begin streaming in seconds. But experts caution that instant gratification comes at a price: It's making us less patient."

Research shows that unless a website or video loads on our smart device in two seconds, we start moving on to other sites. If it takes five seconds, 25% of us leave and if it takes ten seconds, 50% of us leave the site. We want it instantly.

In the space below, name a time when you were impatient.

_____

_____

Like Sarai, our impatience makes us choose poorly. We try a fad diet because it promises quick weight loss. We believe that if we do this one parenting technique, we'll have a different kid by the end of the week. Sometimes, we are so impatient that our goal is simply to get it done and move on the next place or task.

Now think carefully about the answer to this question. Describe the situation when you know you should have waited on God, and then describe what you did instead of waiting.

_____

_____

Our need for instant gratification creates unhappiness in us because we are constantly searching for more. But the bigger problem is that we try to take over for God especially when we can't wait on Him to act in our behalf. Sarai's problem was that she was impatient with God. She tried to accomplish God's will with her own plan. What did you lose by taking action without waiting on God?

_____

_____

Review the symptoms listed below and circle any that describe your feelings.

Sighing	Sad
Sobbing	Can't Think
Can't Concentrate	Can't Sleep
Sleep too Much	Can't Eat
Eat too Much	Eating is Out of Control
Anger is Out of Control	No Plans for the Future
Don't Feel Anything	Isolating Myself from Others

Whatever your job or income situation is today, can you see God's hand working in your life? Be specific?

_____

_____

CHAPTER TEN: LOST YOUTH

When we are born, we begin aging and we can't stop the clock. But we can prevent the normal losses of aging to devastate us. There is no need to fear the process of aging, and we must not give up living or park ourselves in front of the TV with no hope of the future.

In the list below, circle some of the areas that you've noticed or felt concerned about as you age. Circle at least three.

Loss of Memory	Muscle Loss (Scarcopenia)
Loss of Teeth	Hair Loss or Thinning
Hearing Loss (Presbycusis)	Cognitive Loss
Loss of Strength	Loss of Mobility
Loss of Smell	Loss of Taste
Vision Loss	Loss of Joy

Of the top three that you circled, write a sentence to explain why you fear this loss (for example: *I fear losing my hearing because my mother lost hers as she aged*).

1. _____

2. _____

3. _____

How do you feel about the possibility of each of these age-related losses? Write words that describe your feelings such as afraid, ashamed, sad, angry, etc. and then, rate your feelings on the scale 1-10 with 10 being intense and 1 being mild.

1. Age-Related Fear: _____ My feelings: _____

    1......2......3........4........5......6........7........8......9........10

2. Age-Related Fear: _____ My feelings: _____

    1......2......3........4........5......6........7........8......9........10

3. Age Related Fear: _____ My feelings: _____

    1......2......3........4........5......6........7........8......9........10

Perhaps memory loss is the one age-related fear that frightens us the most because diseases such as Alzheimer's have touched many of our lives. Lapses of memory function is frustrating but it is also normal as we age and not the same as more serious dementia. Asking, "Where are my keys?" or when we can't find our glasses or call someone by the wrong name, we are probably not facing serious dementia because these kinds of lapses are normal. When we come into a room and can't remember why or when, something seems to be on the "tip of my tongue" but we can't recall it, we are experiencing the slowing of the mental processing function, which is not the same as memory loss. Age related temporary memory slips do not affect our ability to carry out a task, nor does it eliminate your wisdom and knowledge and common sense.

> *Note: Some age-related memory losses go beyond the normal slowing of the mental processing function and may develop into Mild Cognitive Impairment (MCI), forgetting appointments, conversations, and being unable to take all the steps necessary to complete a project. MCI is a clinical diagnosis that should be made by a doctor. Dementia or Alzheimer's is also a clinical diagnosis that must be made by a doctor. Symptoms may include forgetting how to do daily tasks such as brushing teeth or washing face or other tasks such as paying bills. A person who is experiencing these symptoms may get lost or disoriented or repeat phrases continuously. With age-related memory problems, you may forget the name of a high school friend, but if you forget the name of your child or spouse, then it might be wise to visit a doctor.*

Scientists are researching constantly to find causes and origins of age-related loss. Listed below are some of the reasons that these researchers are discovering. Look over this list and put a check by the causes that you think might be important to consider.

- ☐ Depression
- ☐ Lack of Exercise
- ☐ Vitamin B12 Deficiency
- ☐ Too Many Calories
- ☐ Thyroid Problems
- ☐ Eating Fatty High Calorie Foods
- ☐ Alcohol Use and Abuse
- ☐ Dehydration
- ☐ Side Effects of Medicine

Experts give many ways we can combat the losses from aging. In the space below each suggestion listed, write your specific plan to slow down or stop the loss from aging.

Stay social, engaging others face-to-face.

_____

_____

Exercise (aerobic, walking, hand-eye coordination games, exercises that use both arms and legs) (According to the American Academy of Neurology, walking 6-9 miles per week can prevent brain shrinkage.)

_____

_____

MYplace O FOR DISCOVERY

Don't Smoke

_____

_____

Control Stress

_____

_____

Regulate Sleep

_____

_____

Eat Fruits and Vegetables

_____

_____

Drink Water

_____

_____

Drink Green Tea

_____

_____

Eat Foods rich in Omega-3 (Salmon, Flax, Tuna, Walnuts, etc)

_____

_____

What "brain exercises" do you think would be helpful to battle the slowing of mental processes? (some suggestions: word games, strategy puzzles, reading, learning a new skill, taking a course, learning a new computer program, photography). Be specific with ideas that you will do.

_____

_____

Why do you think that taking on projects that require planning and follow-through (for example: quilting or building a garden) would be good for brain function?

_____

_____

Research shows that laughter is another important antidote for stimulating your brain. Can you describe why this might be true? Describe the last time you experienced an uncontrollable belly laugh.

_____

_____

Remember laughter includes being able to laugh at yourself. What is one thing about you that makes you smile or laugh?

_____

_____

Including laughter in your life means spending time with people who are fun and enjoyable. How can you make more time for enjoyable friends? How can you avoid those who bring your spirit down?

_____

_____

Aging causes us to feel concerned about our looks. Hairlines recede, ears grow longer, noses drop, eyes bag, chin and jowls sag, and necks wiggle. Wrinkles appear on the forehead, eyebrows, and around our eyes and lips. These facial changes challenge our joy and confidence and sometimes our desire to achieve or persevere. How can you celebrate age and age-related appearance? Be specific.

_____

_____

Physical (sun protection, creams, lotions, medical procedures)

_____

_____

Mental (developing skills that build confidence regardless of age-related appearance)

_____

_____

Emotional (Celebrate achievements, milestones, and accomplishments)

_____

_____

Spiritual (Consider what God has done and how it affects who you are today)

_____

_____

Read Ephesians 2:10. What does this verse say about what God thinks about us?

_____

_____

How does the fact that you are God's workmanship—His hand-crafted creation—help you understand why participation in FP4H is part of your proper response to God's grace?

_____

_____

CHAPTER ELEVEN: CELEBRATION

You've got to be willing to lose everything to gain yourself." – Iyanla Vanzant

Living as a Christ follower is full of paradoxical truth. Jesus said to die is to live and to give is to have. These contradictions seem odd to us, but maybe none so strange as Jesus saying that "To gain is to lose." But if we can grasp the concepts, we discover the key to healthy living.

Loss, though painful in the moment, is transformative if we handle it well and see the loss from God's divine viewpoint. Let's consider what we've learned during this session of *My Place for Discovery*. What new perspective did you gain from looking at the following "losses" through a new lens?

Lost Friendship, Relationship, Love

_____

_____

Lost Possessions

_____

_____

Lost Health

_____

_____

Loss through Death

_____

_____

Lost Dreams & Opportunities

_____

_____

Lost Freedom

_____

_____

Lost Identity

_____

_____

Lost Job

_____

_____

Lost Youth

_____

_____

How has your new perspective on loss helped you to maintain healthy eating habits—without overeating or starving yourself?

_____

_____

What healthy food choices have you made?

_____

_____

Celebrate your new perspective on loss by finding a Scripture verse or an appropriate quote that expresses how you have changed in the following areas.

Spiritually

_____

_____

Emotionally

_____

_____

ELEVEN CELEBRATION

Physically

_____

_____

Mentally.

_____

_____

Write a sentence that expresses how Jesus has helped you face loss in a renewed way.

_____

_____

_____

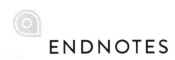

ENDNOTES

[1] Mark Batterson – Draw the Circle: The 40 Day Prayer Challenge, Zondervan, 2012. ibid
[2] Carlin Flora , Friendfluence, Anchor Publishers, 2013, page 6
[3] Joyce Ainsworth, Food, Freedom, and Finish Lines, Used by permission.
[4] http://www.pweathersafety.ohio.gov/Documents/FactSheets/ODMH%20Brochure%20-%20Dealing%20w%20Emotions%20after%20Storm.pdf accessed May 2016
[5] Cynthia Ruchti, Song of Silence, Abington Press, 2016.
[6] Ainsworth, Used by permission
[7] adapted from article Traumatic Stress, http://www.helpguide.org/articles/ptsd-trauma/traumatic-stress.htm accessed June 2016
[8] https://healthcare.utah.edu/huntsmancancerinstitute/cancer-information/resources/factsheetpdfs/grieflossofhealth.pdf
[9] https://www.bostonglobe.com/lifestyle/style/2013/02/01/the-growing-culture-impatience-where-instant-gratification-makes-crave-more-instant-gratification/q8tWDNGeJB2mm45fQxtTQP/story.html accessed October 2016

Made in the USA
Columbia, SC
21 May 2024